A Beginner Guide to Your Keto Chaffle Meals

Quick and Easy Meat Recipes to Boost Your Metabolism

Kade Harrison

Table of Contents

Grill Beefsteak And Chaffle

Preparation Time:

5 minutes

Cooking Time:

10 minutes

Servings: 1

Ingredients:

- 1 beefsteak rib eye
- 1 tsp salt
- 1 tsp pepper
- 1 tbsp. lime juice
- 1 tsp garlic

Directions:

1. Prepare your grill for direct heat.
2. Mix together all spices and rub over beefsteak evenly.
3. Place the beef on the grill rack over medium heat.
4. Cover and cook steak for about6 to 8 minutes. Flip and cook for another 4-5 minutes until cooked through.
5. Serve with keto simple chaffle and enjoy!

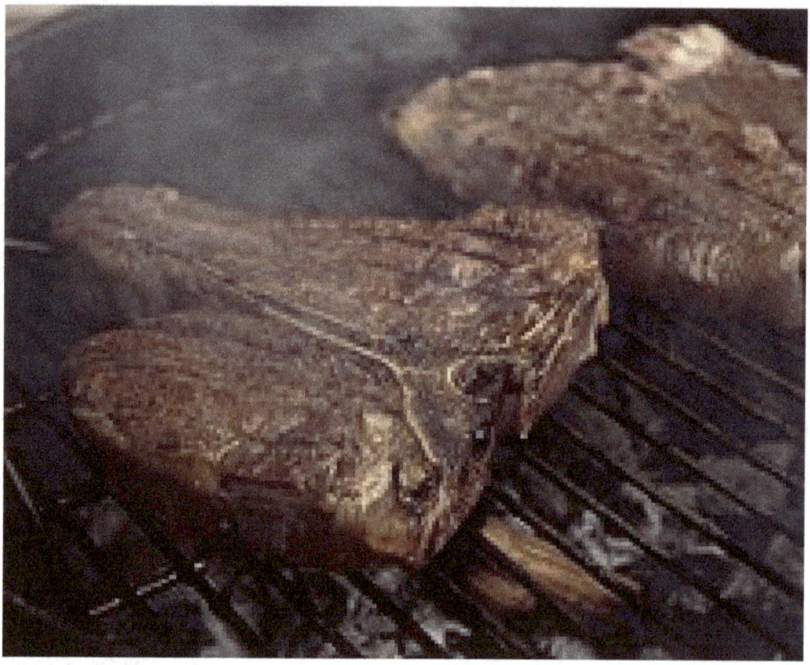

Barbecue Chaffle

Preparation Time:

5 minutes

Cooking Time:

8 minutes

Servings: 2

Ingredients:

- 1 egg, beaten
- ½ cup cheddar cheese, shredded
- ½ teaspoon barbecue sauce
- ¼ teaspoon baking powder

Directions:

1. Plug in your waffle maker to preheat.
2. Mix all the ingredients in a bowl.
3. Pour half of the mixture to your waffle maker.
4. Cover and cook for 4 minutes.
5. Repeat the same steps for the next barbecue chaffle.

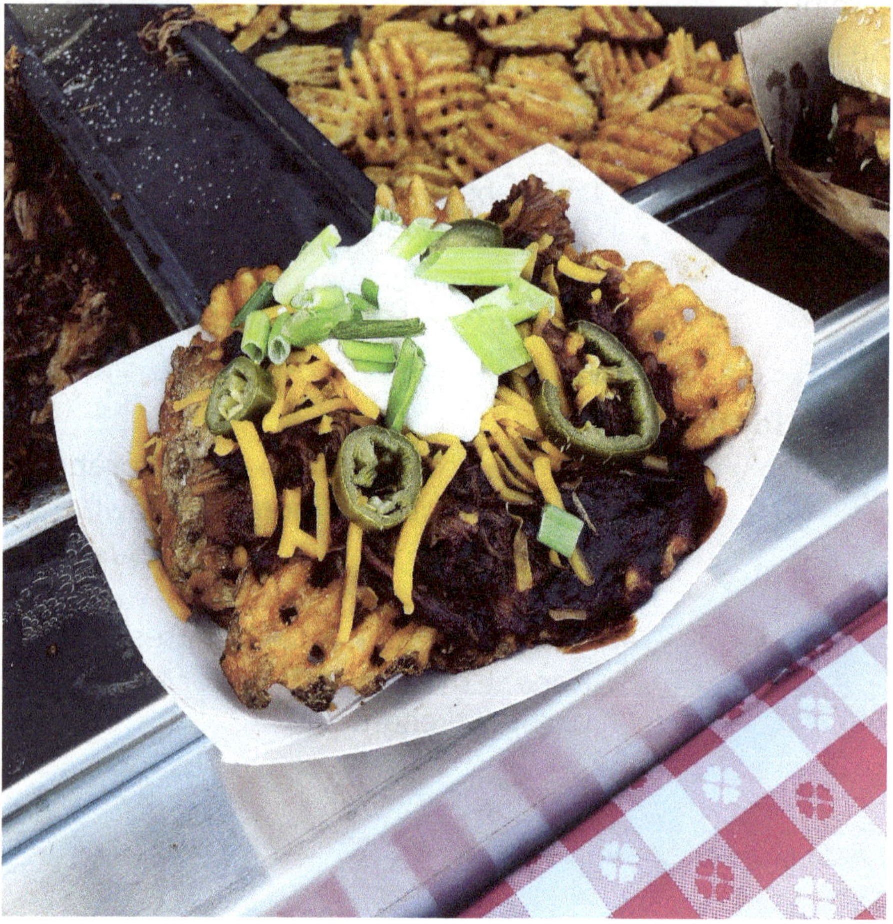

Turkey Chaffle Burger

Preparation Time:

10 minutes

Cooking Time:

10 minutes

Servings: 2

Ingredients:

- 2 cups ground turkey
- Salt and pepper to taste
- 1 tablespoon olive oil
- 4 garlic chaffles
- 1 cup Romaine lettuce, chopped
- 1 tomato, sliced
- Mayonnaise
- Ketchup

Directions:

1. Combine ground turkey, salt and pepper.
2. Form 2 thick burger patties.
3. Add the olive oil to a pan over medium heat.
4. Cook the turkey burger until fully cooked on both sides.
5. Spread mayo on the chaffle.
6. Top with the turkey burger, lettuce and tomato.

7. Squirt ketchup on top before topping with another chaffle.

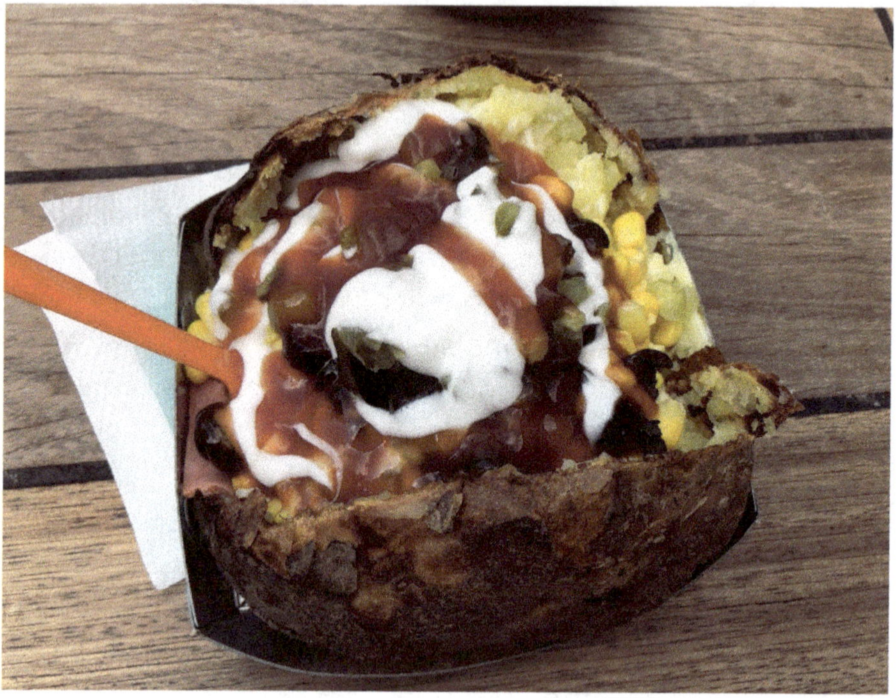

Savory Beef Chaffle

Preparation Time:

10 minutes

Cooking Time:

15 minutes

Servings: 2

Ingredients:

- 1 teaspoon olive oil
- 2 cups ground beef
- Garlic salt to taste
- 1 red bell pepper, sliced into strips
- 1 green bell pepper, sliced into strips
- 1 onion, minced
- 1 bay leaf
- 2 garlic chaffles
- Butter

Directions:

1. Put your pan over medium heat.
2. Add the olive oil and cook ground beef until brown.
3. Season with garlic salt and add bay leaf.
4. Drain the fat, transfer to a plate and set aside.
5. Discard the bay leaf.
6. In the same pan, cook the onion and bell peppers for 2 minutes.
7. Put the beef back to the pan.
8. Heat for 1 minute.

9. Spread butter on top of the chaffle.
10. Add the ground beef and veggies.
11. Roll or fold the chaffle.

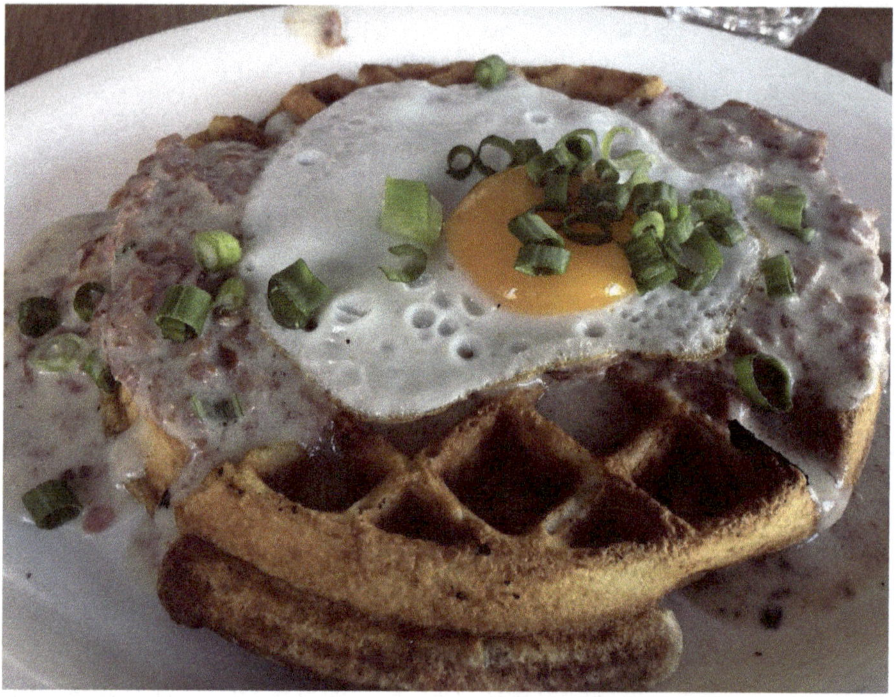

Spicy Shrimp and Chaffles

Preparation Time:

15 minutes

Cooking Time:

31 minutes

Servings: 4

Ingredients:

- For the shrimp:
- 1 tbsp olive oil
- 1 lb jumbo shrimp, peeled and deveined
- 1 tbsp Creole seasoning
- Salt to taste
- 2 tbsp hot sauce
- 3 tbsp butter
- 2 tbsp chopped fresh scallions to garnish
- For the chaffles:
- 2 eggs, beaten
- 1 cup finely grated Monterey Jack cheese

Directions:

1. For the shrimp:
2. Heat the olive oil in a medium skillet over medium heat.
3. Season the shrimp with the Creole seasoning and salt. Cook in the oil until pink and opaque on both sides, 2 minutes.

4. Pour in the hot sauce and butter. Mix well until the shrimp is adequately coated in the sauce, 1 minute.
5. Turn the heat off and set aside.
6. For the chaffles:
7. Preheat the waffle iron.
8. In a medium bowl, mix the eggs and Monterey Jack cheese.
9. Open the iron and add a quarter of the mixture. Close and cook until crispy, 7 minutes.
10. Transfer the chaffle to a plate and make 3 more chaffles in the same manner.
11. Cut the chaffles into quarters and place on a plate.
12. Top with the shrimp and garnish with the scallions.
13. Serve warm.

Chicken Jalapeño Chaffles

Preparation Time:

15 minutes

Cooking Time:

14 minutes

Servings: 2

Ingredients:

- 1/8 cup finely grated Parmesan cheese
- ¼ cup finely grated cheddar cheese
- 1 egg, beaten
- ½ cup cooked chicken breasts, diced
- 1 small jalapeño pepper, deseeded and minced
- 1/8 tsp garlic powder
- 1/8 tsp onion powder
- 1 tsp cream cheese, softened

Directions:

1. Preheat the waffle iron.
2. In a medium bowl, mix all the ingredients until adequately combined.
3. Open the iron and add half of the mixture. Close and cook until crispy, 7 minutes.
4. Transfer the chaffle to a plate and make a second chaffle in the same manner.

5. Allow cooling and serve afterward.

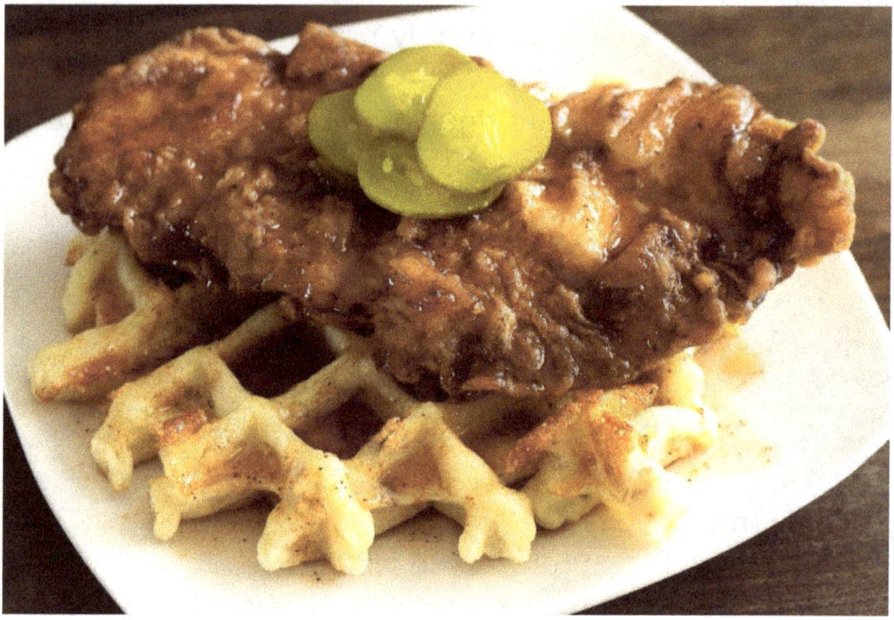

Chicken and Chaffle Nachos

Preparation Time:

15 minutes

Cooking Time:

33 minutes

Servings: 4

Ingredients:

- For the chaffles:
- 2 eggs, beaten
- 1 cup finely grated Mexican cheese blend
- For the chicken-cheese topping:
- 2 tbsp butter
- 1 tbsp almond flour
- ¼ cup unsweetened almond milk
- 1 cup finely grated cheddar cheese + more to garnish
- 3 bacon slices, cooked and chopped
- 2 cups cooked and diced chicken breasts
- 2 tbsp hot sauce
- 2 tbsp chopped fresh scallions

Directions:

1. For the chaffles:
2. Preheat the waffle iron.
3. In a medium bowl, mix the eggs and Mexican cheese blend.
4. Open the iron and add a quarter of the mixture. Close and cook until crispy, 7 minutes.

5. Transfer the chaffle to a plate and make 3 more chaffles in the same manner.
6. Place the chaffles on serving plates and set aside for serving.
7. For the chicken-cheese topping:
8. Melt the butter in a large skillet and mix in the almond flour until brown, 1 minute.
9. Pour the almond milk and whisk until well combined. Simmer until thickened, 2 minutes.
10. Stir in the cheese to melt, 2 minutes and then mix in the bacon, chicken, and hot sauce.
11. Spoon the mixture onto the chaffles and top with some more cheddar cheese.
12. Garnish with the scallions and serve immediately.

Buffalo Hummus Beef Chaffles

Preparation Time:

15 minutes

Cooking Time:

32 minutes

Servings: 4

Ingredients:

- 2 eggs
- 1 cup + ¼ cup finely grated cheddar cheese, divided
- 2 chopped fresh scallions
- Salt and freshly ground black pepper to taste
- 2 chicken breasts, cooked and diced
- ¼ cup buffalo sauce
- 3 tbsp low-carb hummus
- 2 celery stalks, chopped
- ¼ cup crumbled blue cheese for topping

Directions:

1. Preheat the waffle iron.
2. In a medium bowl, mix the eggs, 1 cup of the cheddar cheese, scallions, salt, and black pepper,
3. Open the iron and add a quarter of the mixture. Close and cook until crispy, 7 minutes.
4. Transfer the chaffle to a plate and make 3 more chaffles in the same manner.

5. Preheat the oven to 400 F and line a baking sheet with parchment paper. Set aside.
6. Cut the chaffles into quarters and arrange on the baking sheet.
7. In a medium bowl, mix the chicken with the buffalo sauce, hummus, and celery.
8. Spoon the chicken mixture onto each quarter of chaffles and top with the remaining cheddar cheese.
9. Place the baking sheet in the oven and bake until the cheese melts, 4 minutes.
10. Remove from the oven and top with the blue cheese.
11. Serve afterward.

Pork Rind Chaffle

Preparation time:

10 minutes

Cooking time:

20 minutes

Servings: 4 medium chaffles

Ingredients:

- 1 1/3 cup / 150 grams shredded mozzarella cheese
- 4 eggs, at room temperature
- 2 cups / 475 grams crushed pork rinds
- Sour cream for topping

Directions:

1. Take a non-stick waffle iron, plug it in, select the medium or medium-high heat setting and let it preheat until ready to use; it could also be indicated with an indicator light changing its color.
2. Meanwhile, prepare the batter, and for this, place pork rind in a food processor and process for 1 minute until mixture resembles grains.
3. Take a large bowl, crack eggs in it, add pork rinds and cheese, and mix with a hand whisk until smooth.
4. Use a ladle to pour one-fourth of the prepared batter into the heated waffle iron in a spiral direction, starting from the edges, then shut

the lid and cook for 5 minutes or more until solid and nicely browned; the cooked waffle will look like a cake.

5. When done, transfer chaffles to a plate with a silicone spatula and repeat with the remaining batter.
6. Let chaffles stand for some time until crispy, top with a dollop of sour cream and serve.

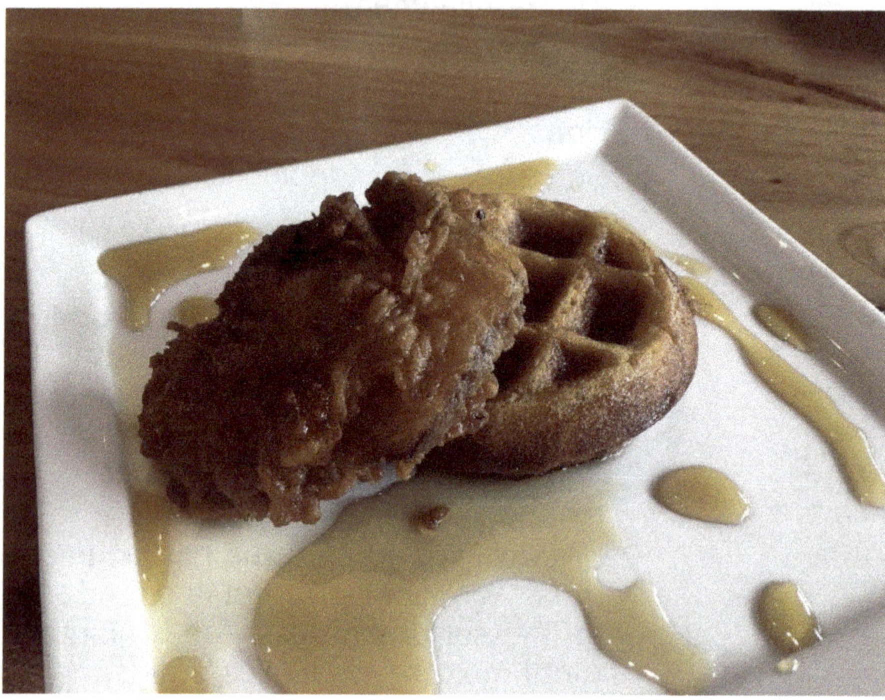

Cheesy Chicken and Ham Chaffle

Preparation time:

5 minutes

Cooking time:

12 minutes

Servings: 4 mini chaffles

Ingredients:

- 4 tablespoons chopped ham
- 1/4 cup / 60 grams diced chicken, cooked
- 1/4 cup / 30 grams shredded Swiss cheese
- 1 egg, at room temperature
- 1/4 cup / 30 grams shredded mozzarella cheese

Directions:

1. Take a non-stick mini waffle iron, plug it in, select the medium or medium-high heat setting and let it preheat until ready to use; it could also be indicated with an indicator light changing its color.
2. Meanwhile, prepare the batter and for this, take a large bowl, crack eggs in it, beat with a hand whisk, then add remaining ingredients and whisk until incorporated.
3. Use a ladle to pour one-fourth of the prepared batter into the heated waffle iron in a spiral direction, starting from the edges, then shut

the lid and cook for 4 minutes or more until solid and nicely browned; the cooked waffle will look like a cake.

4. When done, transfer chaffles to a plate with a silicone spatula and repeat with the remaining batter.
5. Let chaffles stand for some time until crispy and serve straight away.

Cloud Bread Cheddar Chaffle

Preparation time:

10 minutes

Cooking time:

20 minutes

Servings: 4

Ingredients:

- ¼ cup / 60 grams whey protein powder
- ¼ teaspoon salt
- ½ teaspoon baking powder
- ¼ cup / 60 grams sour cream
- ½ cup / 55 shredded cheddar cheese
- 3 eggs, at room temperature
- Crispy bacon for topping
- Chopped chives for topping

Directions:

1. Take a non-stick waffle iron, plug it in, select the medium or medium-high heat setting and let it preheat until ready to use; it could also be indicated with an indicator light changing its color.
2. Meanwhile, prepare the batter and for this, take a large bowl, crack eggs in it, add remaining ingredients except for the toppings and then stir with an electric mixer until smooth.
3. Use a ladle to pour one-fourth of the prepared batter into the heated

waffle iron in a spiral direction, starting from the edges, then shut the lid and cook for 5 minutes or more until solid and nicely browned; the cooked waffle will look like a cake.

4. When done, transfer chaffles to a plate with a silicone spatula and repeat with the remaining batter.
5. Let chaffles stand for some time until crispy, then top with bacon, sprinkle with chives, and serve straight away.

Corn Bread Chaffle

Preparation time:

10 minutes

Cooking time:

20 minutes

Servings: 4 medium chaffles

Ingredients:

- 3 cups / 290 grams ground almonds, blanched
- 2 teaspoons baking soda
- 8 tablespoons hemp seeds
- 1 teaspoon baking powder
- 1 teaspoon of sea salt
- 4 tablespoons avocado oil
- 8 tablespoons coconut milk, unsweetened
- 4 eggs, at room temperature

Directions:

1. Take a non-stick waffle iron, plug it in, select the medium or medium-high heat setting and let it preheat until ready to use; it could also be indicated with an indicator light changing its color.
2. Meanwhile, prepare the batter and for this, take a large bowl, add almonds and seeds in it and then stir in salt, baking powder, and soda until combined.

3. Take a separate bowl, crack eggs in it, add oil, pour in milk, stir with a hand whisk until frothy, and then stir this mixture with a spoon into the almond mixture until incorporated.
4. Use a ladle to pour one-fourth of the prepared batter into the heated waffle iron in a spiral direction, starting from the edges, then shut the lid and cook for 5 minutes or more until solid and nicely browned; the cooked waffle will look like a cake.
5. When done, transfer chaffles to a plate with a silicone spatula and repeat with the remaining batter.
6. Let chaffles stand for some time until crispy and serve straight away.

Brie, Basil and Tomato Chaffle

Preparation time:

10 minutes

Cooking time:

24 minutes

Servings: 4 mini chaffles

Ingredients:

- 4 cherry tomatoes, diced
- 1 teaspoon dried basil
- 1 cup / 235 grams Brie cheese cubes, softened
- 2 eggs, at room temperature

Directions:

1. Take a non-stick mini waffle iron, plug it in, select the medium or medium-high heat setting and let it preheat until ready to use; it could also be indicated with an indicator light changing its color.
2. Meanwhile, prepare the batter and for this, take a large bowl, crack eggs in it, add cheese, tomatoes, and basil and mix with a hand whisk until combined.
3. Use a ladle to pour one-fourth of the prepared batter into the heated waffle iron in a spiral direction, starting from the edges, then shut the lid and cook for 4 to 6 minutes until solid and nicely browned; the cooked waffle will look like a cake.

4. When done, transfer chaffles to a plate with a silicone spatula and repeat with the remaining batter.
5. Let chaffles stand for some time until crispy and serve straight away.

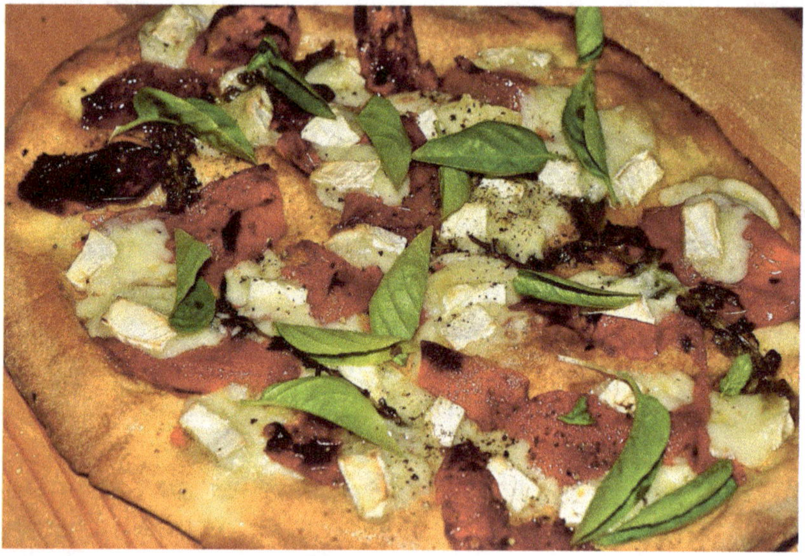

Broccoli Chaffle

Preparation time:

10 minutes

Cooking time:

15 minutes

Servings: 3 medium chaffles

Ingredients:

- 1 cup / 175 grams broccoli florets
- 2 eggs, at room temperature
- 6 tablespoons grated parmesan cheese
- 1 cup / 115 grams shredded cheddar cheese

Directions:

1. Take a non-stick waffle iron, plug it in, select the medium or medium-high heat setting and let it preheat until ready to use; it could also be indicated with an indicator light changing its color.
2. Meanwhile, prepare the batter, and for this, place broccoli florets in a blender and pulse for 1 to 2 minutes until florets resemble rice.
3. Tip the broccoli in a medium bowl, add remaining ingredients and then stir with a hand whisk until combined.
4. Use a ladle to pour one-third of the prepared batter into the heated waffle iron in a spiral direction,

starting from the edges, then shut the lid and cook for 5 minutes or more until solid and nicely browned; the cooked waffle will look like a cake.

5. When done, transfer chaffles to a plate with a silicone spatula and repeat with the remaining batter.
6. Let chaffles stand for some time until crispy and serve straight away.

Cheesy Spinach Chaffle

Preparation time:

10 minutes

Cooking time:

20 minutes

Servings: 4 large chaffles

Ingredients:

- 1 cup / 225 grams frozen baby spinach, thawed
- ½ teaspoon ground black pepper
- ½ teaspoon salt
- ½ teaspoon cumin
- 1 cup / 115 grams grated cheddar cheese
- 8 eggs, at room temperature
- For the Avocado Sauce:
- 1 medium avocado, pitted, diced
- ¼ teaspoon ground black pepper
- 1/3 teaspoon salt
- 2 limes, juiced
- 2 tablespoons coconut milk, unsweetened

Directions:

1. Take a non-stick waffle iron, plug it in, select the medium or medium-high heat setting and let it preheat until ready to use; it could also be indicated with an indicator light changing its color.

2. Meanwhile, prepare the batter for the chaffles, and for this, squeeze moisture from the spinach in a fine sieve as much as possible and then chop it.
3. Take a large bowl, add spinach in it along with cheese, cumin, black pepper, salt and eggs, and stir with a hand whisk until smooth.
4. Use a ladle to pour one-fourth of the prepared batter into the heated waffle iron in a spiral direction, starting from the edges, then shut the lid and cook for 5 minutes or more until solid and nicely browned; the cooked waffle will look like a cake.
5. When done, transfer chaffles to a plate with a silicone spatula and repeat with the remaining batter.
6. In the meantime, prepare the sauce, and for this, place diced avocado in a blender along with remaining ingredients and process for 1 minute until smooth.
7. Let chaffles stand for some time until crispy, then drizzle with prepared avocado sauce and serve straight away.

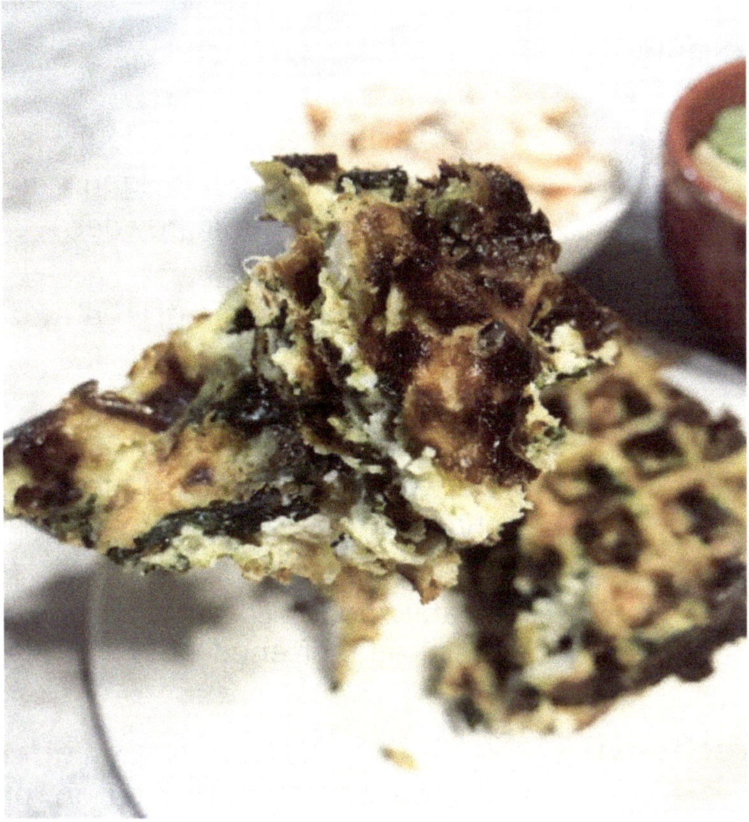

Chaffle Bread Sticks

Preparation time:

10 minutes

Cooking time:

13 minutes

Servings: 2 medium chaffles

Ingredients:

- For Chaffles:
- 2 tablespoons almond flour
- 1/2 teaspoon dried oregano
- 1/2 teaspoon garlic powder
- 1/2 teaspoon salt
- 1/2 cup / 60 grams grated mozzarella cheese
- 1 egg, at room temperature
- For Topping:
- 1/4 cup / 30 grams grated mozzarella cheese
- 1/2 teaspoon garlic powder
- 2 tablespoons coconut butter, unsalted, softened

Directions:

1. Take a non-stick waffle iron, plug it in, select the medium or medium-high heat setting and let it preheat until ready to use; it could also be indicated with an indicator light changing its color.
2. Meanwhile, prepare the batter and for this, take a large bowl, crack the

egg in it, add flour, oregano, garlic powder, salt, and mozzarella cheese and mix with an electric mixer until incorporated.

3. Use a ladle to pour half of the prepared batter into the heated waffle iron in a spiral direction, starting from the edges, then shut the lid and cook for 5 minutes or more until solid and nicely browned; the cooked waffle will look like a cake.
4. When done, transfer chaffles to a plate with a silicone spatula and repeat with the remaining batter.
5. Meanwhile, prepare the topping and for this, take a small bowl, add garlic and butter in it and stir well until combined.
6. Let chaffles stand for some time until crispy, then arrange them on a heatproof tray, and drizzle the topping on top.
7. Preheat the grill over medium-high heat, and when hot, place the tray containing chaffle sticks and grill for 3 minutes until cheese has melted.
8. Serve straight away.

Spinach Artichoke Chaffle with Bacon

Preparation time:

5 minutes

Cooking time:

8 minutes

Servings: 2

Ingredients:

- 4 slices of bacon
- ½ cup chopped spinach
- 1/3 cup marinated artichoke (chopped)
- 1 egg
- ¼ tsp garlic powder
- ¼ tsp smoked paprika
- 2 tbsp cream cheese (softened)
- 1/3 cup shredded mozzarella

Directions:

1. Heat up a frying pan and add the bacon slices. Sear until both sides of the bacon slices are browned. Use a slotted spoon to transfer the bacon to a paper towel line plate to drain.
2. Once the bacon slices are cool, chop them into bits and set aside.
3. Plug the waffle maker to preheat it and spray it with a non-stick cooking spray.
4. In a mixing bowl, combine mozzarella, garlic, paprika, cream cheese and egg.

5. Mix until the ingredients are well combined.
6. Add the spinach, artichoke and bacon bit. Mix until they are well incorporated.
7. Pour an appropriate amount of the batter into the waffle maker and spread the batter to the edges to cover all the holes on the waffle maker.
8. Close the waffle maker and cook 4 minutes or more, according to your waffle maker's settings.
9. After the cooking cycle, use a silicone or plastic utensil to remove the chaffle from the waffle maker.
10. Repeat step 6 to 8 until you have cooked all the batter into chaffles.
11. Serve and top with sour cream as desired.

Lobster Chaffle

Preparation time:

5 minutes

Cooking time:

8 minutes

Servings: 2

Ingredients:

- 1 egg (beaten)
- ½ cup shredded mozzarella cheese
- ¼ tsp garlic powder
- ¼ tsp onion powder
- 1/8 tsp Italian seasoning
- Lobster Filling:
- ½ cup lobster tails (defrosted)
- 1 tbsp mayonnaise
- 1 tsp dried basil
- 1 tsp lemon juice
- 1 tbsp chopped green onion

Directions:

1. Plug the waffle maker to preheat it and spray it with a non-stick cooking spray.
2. In a mixing bowl, combine the mozzarella, Italian seasoning, garlic and onion powder. Add the egg and mix until the ingredients are well combined.
3. Pour an appropriate amount of the batter into the waffle maker and

spread out the batter to cover all the holes on the waffle maker.

4. Close the waffle maker and cook for about 4 minutes or according to your waffle maker's settings.
5. After the cooking cycle, use a plastic or silicone utensil to remove and transfer the chaffle to a wire rack to cool.
6. Repeat step 3 to 5 until you have cooked all the batter into chaffles.
7. For the filling, put the lobster tail in a mixing bowl and add the mayonnaise, basil and lemon juice. Toss until the ingredients are well combine.
8. Fill the chaffles with the lobster mixture and garnish with chopped green onion.
9. Serve and enjoy.

Savory Pork Rind Chaffle

Preparation time:

5 minutes

Cooking time:

10 minutes

Servings: 2

Ingredients:

- ¼ tsp paprika
- ¼ tsp oregano
- ¼ tsp garlic powder
- 1/8 tsp ground black pepper or to taste
- ½ onion (finely chopped)
- ½ cup pork rind (crushed)
- ½ cup mozzarella cheese
- 1 large egg (beaten)

Directions:

1. Plug the waffle maker to preheat it and spray I with a non-stick cooking spray.
2. In a mixing bowl, combine the crushed pork rind, cheese, onion, paprika, garlic powder and pepper. Add the egg and mix until the ingredients are well combined.
3. Pour an appropriate amount of the batter into the waffle maker and spread out the batter to cover all the holes on the waffle maker.

4. Close the waffle maker and cook for about 5 minutes or according to your waffle maker's settings.
5. After the cooking cycle, use a plastic or silicone utensil to remove the chaffle from the waffle maker.
6. Repeat step 3 to 5 until you have cooked all the batter into chaffles.
7. Serve and top with sour cream as desired.

Shrimp Avocado Chaffle Sandwich

Preparation time:

10 minutes

Cooking time:

32 minutes

Servings: 4

Ingredients:

- 2 cups shredded mozzarella cheese
- 4 large eggs
- ½ tsp curry powder
- ½ tsp oregano
- Shrimp Sandwich Filling:
- 1-pound raw shrimp (peeled and deveined)
- 1 large avocado (diced)
- 4 slices cooked bacon
- 2 tbsp sour cream
- ½ tsp paprika
- 1 tsp Cajun seasoning
- 1 tbsp olive oil
- ¼ cup onion (finely chopped)
- 1 red bell pepper (diced)

Directions:

1. Plug the waffle maker to preheat it and spray it with a non-stick cooking spray.
2. Break the eggs into a mixing bowl and beat. Add the cheese, oregano and curry. Mix until the ingredients are well combined.

3. Pour an appropriate amount of the batter into the waffle maker and spread out the batter to the edges to cover all the holes on the waffle maker. This should make 8 mini waffles.
4. Close the waffle maker and cook for about 4 minutes or according to your waffle maker's settings.
5. After the cooking cycle, use a silicone or plastic utensil to remove the chaffle from the waffle maker.
6. Repeat step 3 to 5 until you have cooked all the batter into chaffles.
7. Heat up the olive oil in a large skillet over medium to high heat.
8. Add the shrimp and cook until the shrimp is pink and tender.
9. Remove the skillet from heat and use a slotted spoon to transfer the shrimp to a paper towel lined plate to drain for a few minutes.
10. Put the shrimp in a mixing bowl. Add paprika and Cajun seasoning. Toss until the shrimps are all coated with seasoning.
11. To assemble the sandwich, place one chaffle on a flat surface and spread some sour cream over it. Layer some shrimp, onion, avocado, diced pepper and one slice of bacon over it. Cover with another chaffle.
12. Repeat step 10 until you have assembled all the ingredients into sandwiches.

13. Serve and enjoy.

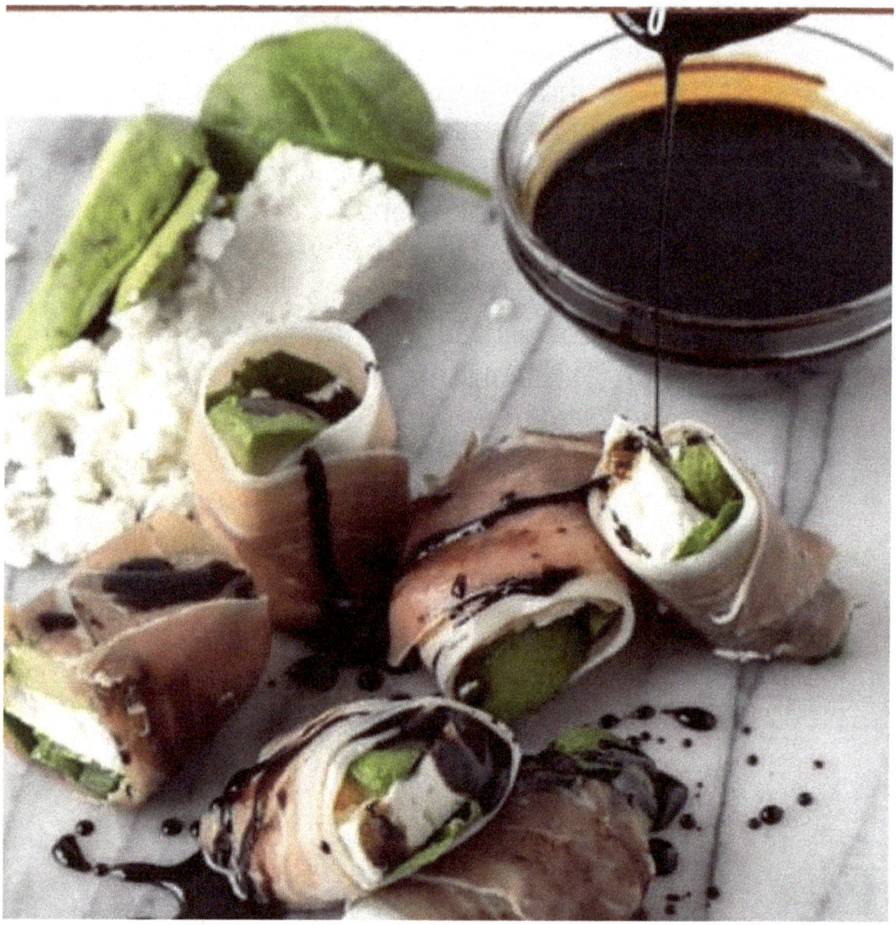

Keto Protein Chaffle

Preparation time:

5 minutes

Cooking time:

8 minutes

Servings: 1

Ingredients:

- 1 egg (beaten)
- ½ cup whey protein powder
- A pinch of salt
- 1 tsp baking powder
- 3 tbsp sour cream
- ½ tsp vanilla extract
- Topping:
- 2 tbsp heavy cream
- 1 tbsp granulated swerve

Directions:

1. Plug the waffle maker to preheat it and spray it with a non-stick cooking spray.
2. In a mixing bowl, whisk together the egg, vanilla and sour cream.
3. In another mixing bowl, combine the protein powder, baking powder and salt.
4. Pour the flour mixture into the egg mixture and mix until the ingredients are well combined and you form a smooth batter.

5. Pour an appropriate amount of the batter into the waffle maker and spread the batter to the edges to cover all the holes on the waffle maker.
6. Close the waffle maker and cook for about 4 minutes or according to your waffle maker's settings.
7. After the cooking cycle, use a plastic or silicone utensil to remove the chaffle from the waffle iron.
8. Repeat step 4 to 6 until you have cooked all the batter into chaffles.
9. For the topping, whisk together the cream and swerve in a mixing bowl until smooth and fluffy.
10. Top the chaffles with the cream and enjoy.

Cauliflower Hash Brown Chaffle

Preparation time:

10 minutes

Cooking time:

8 minutes

Servings: 2

Ingredients:

- 1 egg
- ½ cup cauliflower rice
- ¼ tsp onion powder
- ¼ tsp salt
- ½ tsp garlic powder
- 4 tbsp shredded cheddar cheese
- 1 green onion (chopped)

Directions:

1. Put the cauliflower rice in a microwave safe dish and cover the dish. Place the dish in the microwave and microwave for 3 minutes.
2. Remove the dish from the microwave and stir. Return it to the microwave and steam for about 1 minute or until tender.
3. Let the steamed cauliflower cool for a few minutes. Wrap the steamed cauliflower in a clean towel and squeeze it to remove excess water.
4. Plug the waffle maker to preheat it and spray it with a non-stick cooking spray.

5. In a mixing bowl, combine the cauliflower, green onion, onion powder, cheese, salt, garlic and salt. Add the egg and mix until the ingredients are well combined.
6. Fill your waffle maker with an appropriate amount of the batter and spread out the batter to cover all the holes on the waffle maker.
7. Close the waffle maker and cook until the chaffle is browned. This will take about 4 minutes or more depending on your waffle maker.
8. After the cooking cycle, use a plastic or silicone utensil to remove the chaffle from the waffle maker.
9. Repeat step 6 to 8 until you have cooked all the batter into waffles.
10. Serve the hash brown chaffles and top with your desired topping.

Shirataki Rice Chaffle

Preparation time:

5 minutes

Cooking time:

20 minutes

Servings: 4

Ingredients:

- 2 tbsp almond flour
- ½ tsp oregano
- 1 bag of shirataki rice
- 1 tsp baking powder
- 1 cup shredded cheddar cheese
- 2 eggs (beaten)

Directions:

1. Rinse the shirataki rice with warm water for about 30 seconds and rinse it.
2. Plug the waffle maker to preheat it and spray it with a non-stick cooking spray.
3. In a mixing bowl, combine the rinsed rice, almond flour, baking powder, oregano and shredded cheese.
4. Add the eggs and mix until the ingredients are well combined.
5. Fill the waffle maker with an appropriate amount of the batter and spread out the batter to the edges to cover all the holes on the waffle maker.

6. Close the waffle make and cook for about 5 minutes or according to you waffle maker's settings.
7. After the cooking cycle, use a silicone or plastic utensil to remove the chaffles from the waffle maker.
8. Repeat step 4 to 6 until you have cooked all the batter into chaffles.
9. Serve and enjoy.

Savory Chaffle Stick

Preparation time:

10 minutes

Cooking time:

25 minutes

Servings: 16

Ingredients:

- 6 eggs
- 2 cups shredded mozzarella cheese
- A pinch of salt
- ½ tsp ground black pepper or to taste
- ½ tsp baking powder
- 4 tbsp coconut flour
- 1 tsp onion powder
- 1 tsp garlic powder
- 1 tsp oregano
- ¼ tsp Italian seasoning
- 1 tbsp olive oil
- 1 tbsp melted butter

Directions:

1. Plug the waffle maker to preheat it and spray it with a non-stick cooking spray.
2. Break 4 of the eggs into a mixing bowl and beat.
3. Add the coconut flour, baking powder, salt, cheese and Italian seasoning. Combine until the ingredients are well combined.

4. Add more flour if the mixture is too thick.
5. Pour an appropriate amount of the batter into the waffle maker and spread out the batter to cover all the holes on the waffle maker.
6. Cover the waffle maker and cook for about 7 minutes or according to your waffle maker's settings. Make sure the chaffle is browned.
7. After the cooking cycle, use a plastic or silicone utensil to remove the chaffle form the waffle maker.
8. Repeat step 3 to 5 until you have cooked all the batter into chaffles.
9. Cut the chaffles into sticks. Each mini chaffle should make about 4 sticks.
10. Preheat the oven to 350°F. Line a baking sheet with parchment paper and grease it with the melted butter.
11. Break the remaining two eggs into another mixing bowl and beat.
12. In another mixing bowl, combine the oregano, pepper, garlic and onion.
13. Dip one chaffle stick into the egg. Bring it out and hold it for a few seconds to allow excess liquid to drip off.
14. Dip the wet chaffle stick into the seasoning mixture and make sure it is coated with seasoning. Drop it on the baking sheet.

15. Repeat step 11 and 12 until all the chaffle sticks are coated.
16. Arrange the chaffle sticks into the baking sheet in a single layer.
17. Place the baking sheet in the oven and bake for 10 minutes.
18. Remove the baking sheet from the oven, brush the oil over the sticks and flip them.
19. Return it to the oven and bake for an additional 6 minutes or until the stick are golden brown.
20. Remove the sticks from the oven and let them cool for a few minutes.
21. Serve and enjoy.

Cinnamon Roll Chaffle

Preparation time:

7 minutes

Cooking time:

9 minutes

Servings: 3

Ingredients:

- 1 egg (beaten)
- ½ cup shredded mozzarella cheese
- 1 tsp cinnamon
- 1 tsp sugar free maple syrup
- ¼ tsp baking powder
- 1 tbsp almond flour
- ½ tsp vanilla extract
- Topping:
- 2 tsp granulated swerve
- 1 tbsp heavy cream
- 4 tbsp cream cheese

Directions:

1. Plug the waffle maker to preheat it and spray it with a non-stick spray.
2. In a mixing bowl, whisk together the egg, maple syrup and vanilla extract.
3. In another mixing bowl, combine the cinnamon, almond flour, baking powder and mozzarella cheese.
4. Pour in the egg mixture into the flour mixture and mix until the ingredients are well combined.

5. Pour in an appropriate amount of the batter into the waffle maker and spread out the batter to the edges to cover all the holes on the waffle maker.
6. Close the waffle maker and bake for about 3 minute or according to your waffle maker's settings.
7. After the cooking cycle, use a silicone or plastic utensil to remove the chaffle from the waffle maker.
8. Repeat step 5 to 7 until you have cooked all the batter into chaffles.
9. For the topping, combine the cream cheese, swerve and heavy cream in a microwave safe dish.
10. Place the dish in a microwave and microwave on high until the mixture is melted and smooth. Stir every 15 seconds.
11. Top the chaffles with the cream mixture and enjoy.

Cereal and walnut Chaffle

Preparation time:

5 minutes

Cooking time:

6 minutes

Servings: 2

Ingredients:

- 1 milliliter of cereal flavoring
- ¼ tsp baking powder
- 1 tsp granulated swerve
- 1/8 tsp xanthan gum
- 1 tbsp butter (melted)
- ½ tsp coconut flour
- 2 tbsp toasted walnut (chopped)
- 1 tbsp cream cheese
- 2 tbsp almond flour
- 1 large egg (beaten)
- ¼ tsp cinnamon
- 1/8 tsp nutmeg

Directions:

1. Plug the waffle maker to preheat it and spray it with a non-stick spray.
2. In a mixing bowl, whisk together the egg, cereal flavoring, cream cheese and butter.
3. In another mixing bowl, combine the coconut flour, almond flour, cinnamon, nutmeg, swerve, xanthan gum and baking powder.

4. Pour the egg mixture into the flour mixture and mix until you form a smooth batter.
5. Fold in the chopped walnuts.
6. Pour in an appropriate amount of the batter into the waffle maker and spread out the batter to the edges to cover all the holes on the waffle maker.
7. Close the waffle maker and cook for about 3 minutes or according to your waffle maker's settings.
8. After the cooking cycle, use a plastic or silicone utensil to remove the chaffle from the waffle maker.
9. Repeat step 6 to 8 until you have cooked all the batter into chaffles.
10. Serve and top with sour cream or heavy cream.

Beef Zucchini Chaffle

Preparation time:

10 minutes

Cooking time:

5 minutes

Servings: 2

Ingredients:

- Zucchini: 1 (small)
- Beef: ½ cup boneless
- Egg: 1
- Shredded mozzarella: half cup
- Pepper: as per your taste
- Salt: as per your taste
- Basil: 1 tsp

Directions:

1. Boil beef in water to make it tender
2. Shred it into small pieces and set aside
3. Preheat your waffle iron
4. Grate zucchini finely
5. Add all the ingredients to zucchini in a bowl and mix well
6. Now add the shredded beef
7. Grease your waffle iron lightly
8. Pour the mixture into a full-size waffle maker and spread evenly
9. Cook till it turns crispy
10. Make as many chaffles as your mixture and waffle maker allow

11. Serve crispy and with your favorite keto sauce

Spinach Beef Chaffle

Preparation time:

10 minutes

Cooking time:

5 minutes

Servings: 2

Ingredients:

- Spinach: ½ cup
- Beef: ½ cup boneless
- Egg: 1
- Shredded mozzarella: half cup
- Pepper: as per your taste
- Garlic powder: 1 tbsp
- Salt: as per your taste
- Basil: 1 tsp

Directions:

1. Boil beef in water to make it tender
2. Shred it into small pieces and set aside
3. Boil spinach in a saucepan for 10 minutes and strain
4. Preheat your waffle iron
5. Add all the ingredients to boiled spinach in a bowl and mix well
6. Now add the shredded beef
7. Grease your waffle iron lightly
8. Pour the mixture into a full-size waffle maker and spread evenly
9. Cook till it turns crispy

10. Make as many chaffles as your mixture and waffle maker allow
11. Serve crispy and with your favorite keto sauce

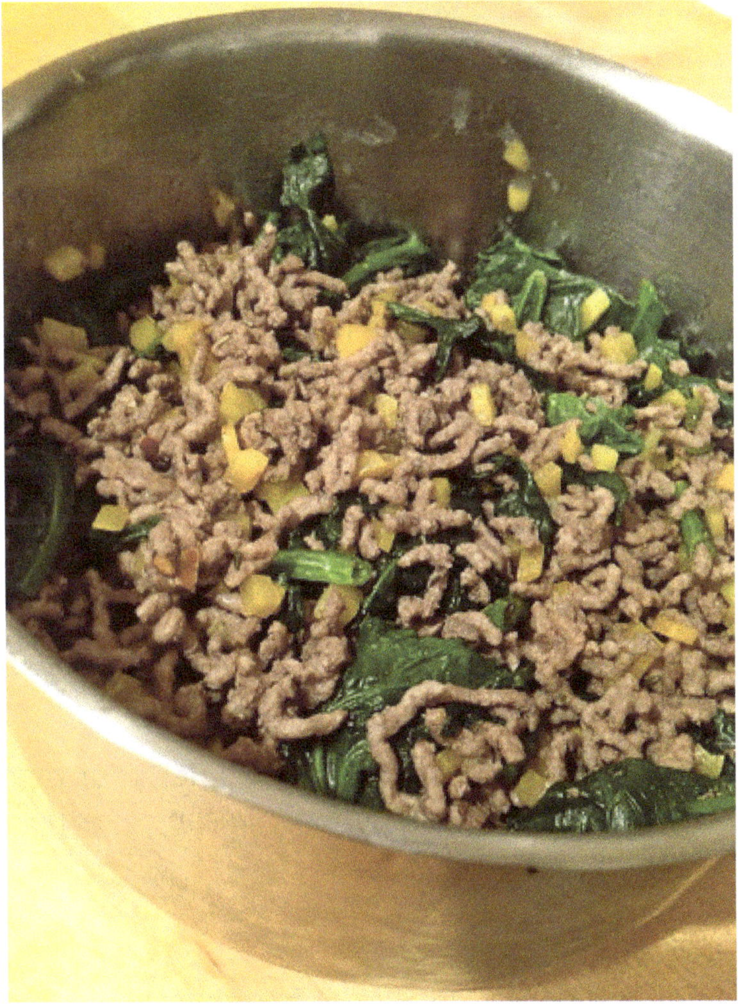

Crispy Beef Burger Chaffle

Preparation time:

20 minutes

Cooking time:

10 minutes

Servings: 2

Ingredients:

- For the chaffle:
- Egg: 2
- Mozzarella cheese: 1 cup (shredded)
- Butter: 1 tbsp
- Almond flour: 2 tbsp
- Baking powder: ¼ tsp
- Onion powder: a pinch
- Garlic powder: a pinch
- Salt: a pinch
- For the beef:
- Ground beef: 1 lb
- Chives: 2 tbsp
- Cheddar cheese: 1 cup
- Salt: ¼ tsp or as per your taste
- Black pepper: ¼ tsp or as per your taste

Directions:

1. Mix all the beef ingredient in a bowl
2. Make patties either grill them or fry them
3. Preheat a mini waffle maker if needed and grease it

4. In a mixing bowl, add all the chaffle ingredients and mix well
5. Pour the mixture to the lower plate of the waffle maker and spread it evenly to cover the plate properly and close the lid
6. Cook for at least 4 minutes to get the desired crunch
7. Remove the chaffle from the heat and keep aside for around one minute
8. Make as many chaffles as your mixture and waffle maker allow
9. Serve with the beef patties in between two chaffles

Crispy Beef Artichoke Chaffle

Preparation time:

10 minutes

Cooking time:

5 minutes

Servings: 2

Ingredients:

- Beef: ½ cup cooked grounded
- Artichokes: 1 cup chopped
- Egg: 1
- Mozzarella cheese: 1/2 cup (shredded)
- Cream cheese: 1 ounce
- Salt: as per your taste
- Garlic powder: ¼ tsp
- Onion powder: ¼ tsp

Directions:

1. Preheat a mini waffle maker if needed and grease it
2. In a mixing bowl, add all the ingredients
3. Mix them all well
4. Pour the mixture to the lower plate of the waffle maker and spread it evenly to cover the plate properly
5. Close the lid
6. Cook for at least 4 minutes to get the desired crunch

7. Remove the chaffle from the heat and keep aside for around one minute
8. Make as many chaffles as your mixture and waffle maker allow
9. Serve hot with your favorite keto sauce

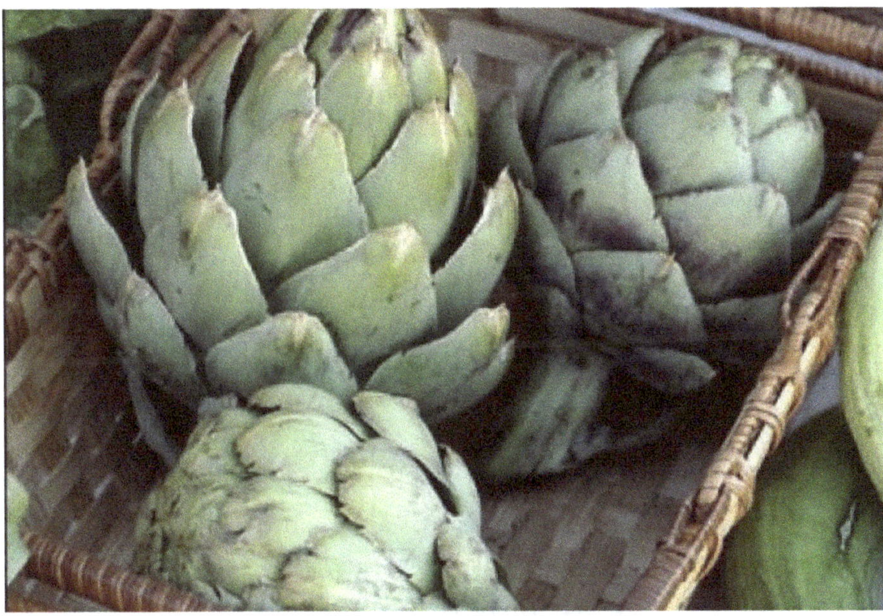

Beef Cheddar Chaffle

Preparation time:

15 minutes

Cooking time:

8 minutes

Servings: 2

Ingredients:

- Beef: 1 cup (grounder)
- Egg: 2
- Chedder cheese: 1 cup
- Mozarrella cheese: 4 tbsp
- Tomato sauce: 6 tbsp
- Basil: ½ tsp
- Garlic: ½ tbsp
- Butter: 1 tsp

Directions:

1. In a pan, add butter and include beef
2. Stir for two minutes and then add garlic and basil
3. Cook till tender
4. Set aside the cooked beef
5. Preheat the mini waffle maker if needed
6. Mix cooked beef, eggs, and 1 cup mozzarella cheese properly
7. Spread it to the mini waffle maker thoroughly
8. Cook for 4 minutes or till it turns crispy and then remove it from the waffle maker

9. Make as many mini chaffles as you can
10. Now in a baking tray, line these mini chaffles and top with the tomato sauce and grated mozzarella cheese
11. Put the tray in the oven at 400 degrees until the cheese melts
12. Serve hot with your favorite keto sauce

Beef Broccoli Chaffle

Preparation time:

10 minutes

Cooking time:

5 minutes

Servings: 2

Ingredients:

- Broccoli: ½ cup
- Beef: ½ cup boneless
- Butter: 2 tbsp
- Egg: 1
- Shredded mozzarella: half cup
- Pepper: as per your taste
- Garlic powder: 1 tbsp
- Salt: as per your taste
- Basil: 1 tsp

Directions:

1. In a pan, add butter and include beef
2. Stir for two minutes and then add garlic and basil
3. Cook till tender
4. Boil broccoli for 10 minutes in a separate pan and blend
5. Set aside the cooked beef
6. Preheat the mini waffle maker if needed
7. Mix cooked beef, broccoli blend, eggs, and 1 cup mozzarella cheese properly

8. Spread it to the mini waffle maker thoroughly
9. Cook for 4 minutes or till it turns crispy and then remove it from the waffle maker
10. Make as many mini chaffles as you can
11. Now in a baking tray, line these mini chaffles and top with the tomato sauce and grated mozzarella cheese
12. Put the tray in the oven at 400 degrees until the cheese melts
13. Serve hot with your favorite keto sauce

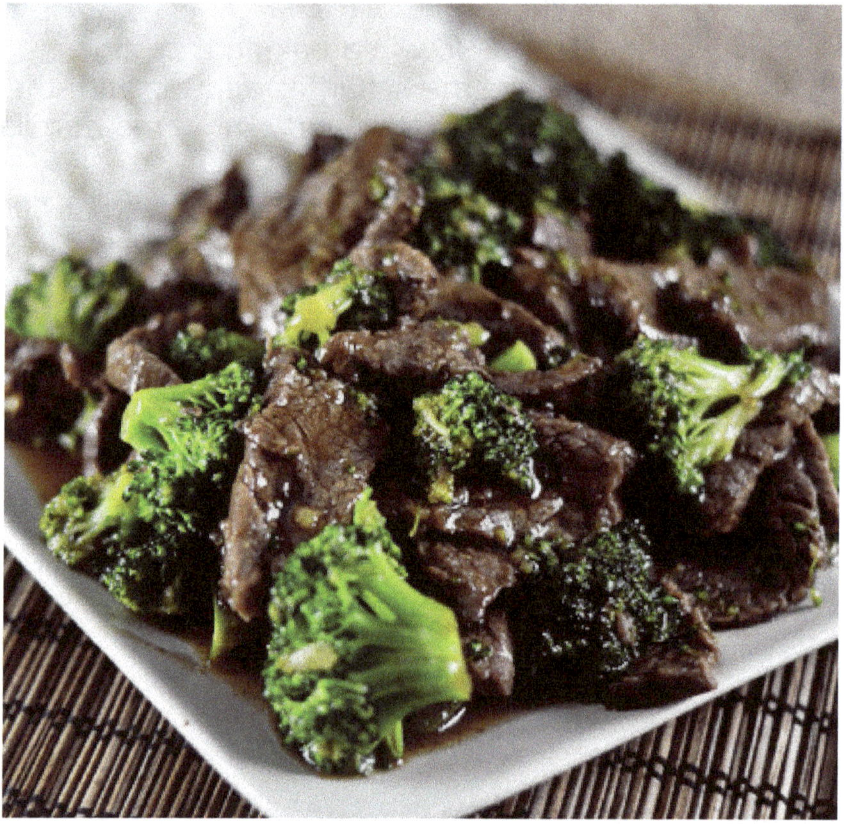

Garlic Lobster Chaffle Roll

Preparation time:

5 minutes

Cooking time:

5 minutes

Servings: 2

Ingredients:

- For chaffle:
- Egg: 2
- Mozzarella cheese: 1 cup (shredded)
- Bay seasoning: ½ tsp
- Garlic powder: ¼ tsp
- For lobster mix:
- Langostino tails: 1 cup
- Kewpie mayo: 2 tbsp
- Garlic powder: ½ tsp
- Lemon juice: 2 tsp
- Parsley: 1 tsp (chopped) for garnishing

Directions:

1. Defrost langostino tails
2. In a small mixing bowl, mix langostino tails with lemon juice, garlic powder, and kewpie mayo; mix properly and keep aside
3. In another mixing bowl, beat eggs and add mozzarella cheese to them with garlic powder and bay seasoning
4. Mix them all well and pour to the greasy mini waffle maker

5. Cook for at least 4 minutes to get the desired crunch
6. Remove the chaffle from the heat, add the lobster mixture in between and fold
7. Make as many chaffles as your mixture and waffle maker allow
8. Serve hot and enjoy!

Fried Fish Chaffles

Preparation time:

15 minutes

Cooking time:

10 minutes

Servings: 2

Ingredients:

- For chaffle:
- Egg: 2
- Mozzarella cheese: 1 cup (shredded)
- Bay seasoning: ½ tsp
- Garlic powder: ¼ tsp
- For fried fish:
- Fish boneless: 1 cup
- Garlic powder: 1 tbsp
- Onion powder: 1 tbsp
- Salt: ¼ tsp or as per your taste
- Black pepper: ¼ tsp or as per your taste
- Turmeric: ¼ tsp
- Red chili flakes: ½ tbsp
- Butter: 2 tbsp

Directions:

1. Marinate the fish with all the ingredients of the fried fish except for butter
2. Melt butter in a medium-size frying pan and add the marinated fish

3. Fry from both sides for at least 5 minutes and set aside
4. Preheat a mini waffle maker if needed and grease it
5. In a mixing bowl, beat eggs and add all the chaffle ingredients
6. Mix them all well
7. Pour the mixture to the lower plate of the waffle maker and spread it evenly to cover the plate properly
8. Close the lid
9. Cook for at least 4 minutes to get the desired crunch
10. Remove the chaffle from the heat and keep aside for around one minute
11. Make as many chaffles as your mixture and waffle maker allow
12. Serve hot with the prepared fish

Crispy Crab Chaffle

Preparation time:

25 minutes

Cooking time:

10 minutes

Servings: 2

Ingredients:

- For chaffle:
- Egg: 1
- Mozzarella cheese: ½ cup (shredded)
- Salt: ¼ tsp or as per your taste
- Black pepper: ¼ tsp or as per your taste
- Ginger powder: 1 tbsp
- For crab
- Crab meat: 1 cup
- Butter: 2 tbsp
- Salt: ¼ tsp or as per your taste
- Black pepper: ¼ tsp or as per your taste
- Red chili flakes: ½ tsp

Directions:

1. In a frying pan, melt butter and fry crab meat for two minutes
2. Add the spices at the end and set aside
3. Mix all the chaffle ingredients well together
4. Pour a thin layer on a preheated waffle iron

5. Add prepared crab and pour again more mixture over the top
6. Cook the chaffle for around 5 minutes
7. Make as many chaffles as your mixture and waffle maker allow
8. Serve hot with your favorite sauce

Simple Cabbage Chaffles

Preparation time:

10 minutes

Cooking time:

5 minutes

Servings: 2

Ingredients:

- Egg: 2
- Mozzarella cheese: 1 cup (shredded)
- Butter: 2 tbsp
- Almond flour: 2 tbsp
- Turmeric: ¼ tsp
- Baking powder: ¼ tsp
- Onion powder: a pinch
- Garlic powder: a pinch
- Salt: as per your taste
- cabbage: 1 cup shredded

Directions:

1. Take a frying pan and melt 1 tbsp of butter
2. Add the shredded cabbage and sauté for 4 minutes and set aside
3. In a mixing bowl, add all the ingredients and mix well
4. Pour a thin layer on a preheated waffle iron
5. Add cabbage on top of the mixture
6. Again add more mixture over the top

7. Cook the chaffle for around 5 minutes
8. Serve hot with your favorite keto sauce

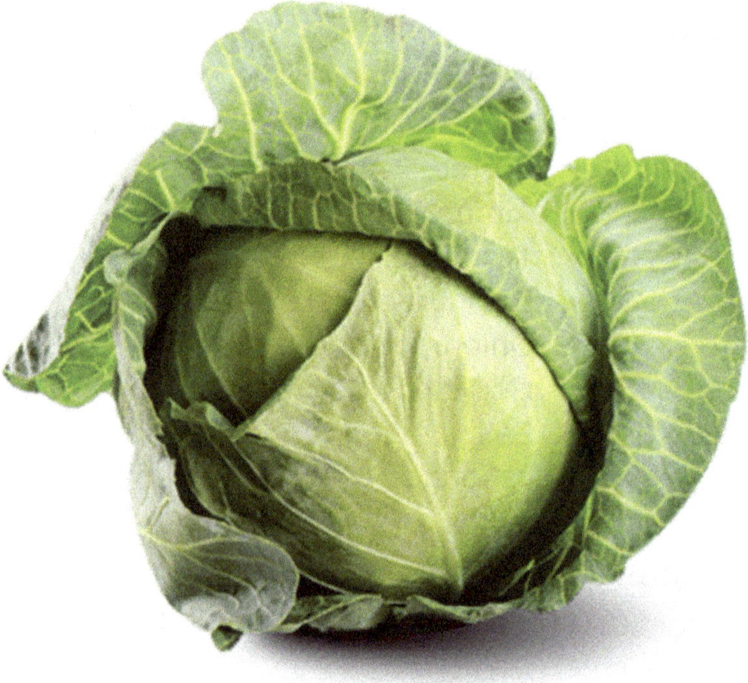

Cabbage and Artichoke Chaffle

Preparation time:

10 minutes

Cooking time:

5 minutes

Servings: 2

Ingredients:

- Artichokes: 1/2 cup chopped
- Cabbage: ½ cup
- Black pepper: ½ tbsp
- Egg: 1
- Mozzarella cheese: 1/2 cup (shredded)
- Cream cheese: 1 ounce
- Salt: as per your taste
- Garlic powder: ¼ tsp
- Turmeric: ¼ tsp
- baking powder: ¼ tsp

Directions:

1. Take a frying pan and melt 1 tbsp of butter
2. Add the shredded cabbage and sauté for 4 minutes and set aside
3. In a mixing bowl, add all the ingredients and mix well
4. Pour a thin layer on a preheated waffle iron
5. Add cabbage on top of the mixture
6. Again add more mixture over the top

7. Cook the chaffle for around 5 minutes
8. Serve hot with your favorite keto sauce

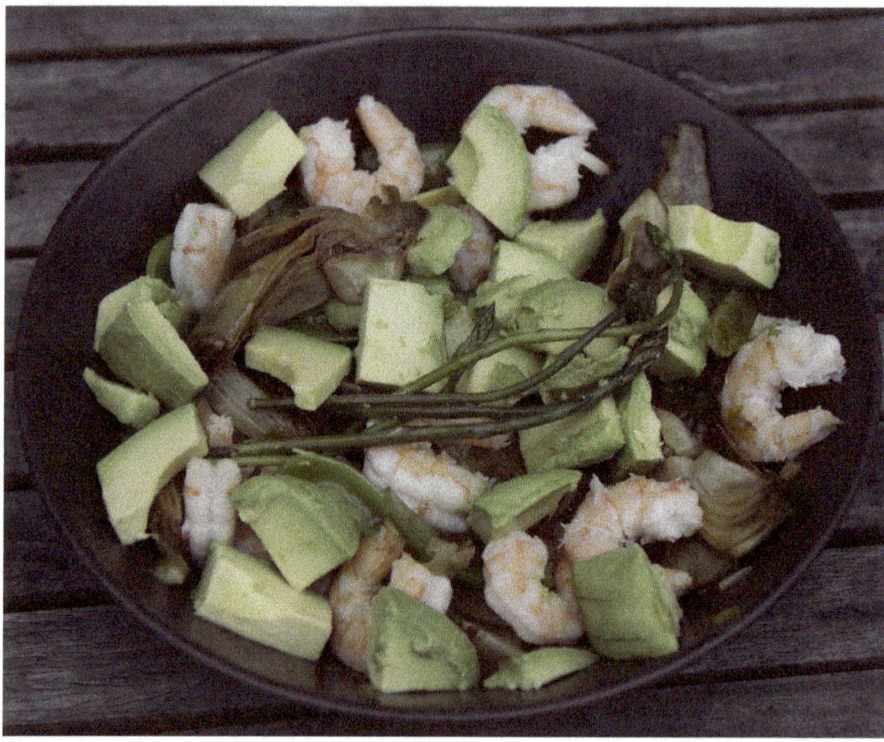

Zucchini BBQ Chaffle

Preparation time:

10 minutes

Cooking time:

5 minutes

Servings: 2

Ingredients:

- Zucchini: 1/2 cup
- Bbq sauce: 1 tbsp (sugar-free)
- Almond flour: 2 tbsp
- Egg: 1
- Cheddar cheese: ½ cup

Directions:

1. Finely grate zucchini
2. Preheat your waffle iron
3. In mixing bowl, add all the chaffle ingredients including zucchini and mix well
4. Grease your waffle iron lightly
5. Pour the mixture to the bottom plate evenly; also spread it out to get better results and close the upper plate and heat
6. Cook for 6 minutes or until the chaffle is done
7. Make as many chaffles as your mixture and waffle maker allow

Eggplant BBQ Chaffle

Preparation time:

10 minutes

Cooking time:

5 minutes

Servings: 2

Ingredients:

- Eggplant: 1/2 cup
- Bbq sauce: 1 tbsp (sugar-free)
- Almond flour: 2 tbsp
- Egg: 1
- cheddar cheese: ½ cup

Directions:

1. Boil egg plant in water, and strain
2. Preheat your waffle iron
3. In mixing bowl, add all the chaffle ingredients including zucchini and mix well
4. Grease your waffle iron lightly
5. Pour the mixture to the bottom plate evenly; also spread it out to get better results and close the upper plate and heat
6. Cook for 6 minutes or until the chaffle is done
7. Make as many chaffles as your mixture and waffle maker allow

Zucchini Olives Chaffles

Preparation time:

10 minutes

Cooking time:

5 minutes

Servings: 2

Ingredients:

- Egg: 2
- Mozzarella cheese: 1 cup (shredded)
- Butter: 1 tbsp
- Almond flour: 2 tbsp
- Turmeric: ¼ tsp
- Baking powder: ¼ tsp
- Onion powder: a pinch
- Garlic powder: a pinch
- Salt: a pinch
- black pepper: ¼ tsp or as per your taste
- spinach: ½ cup
- olives: 5-10

Directions:

1. Boil the spinach in water for around 10 minutes and drain the remaining water
2. In a mixing bowl, add all the above-mentioned ingredients except for olives
3. Mix well and add the boils spinach

4. Pour the mixture to the lower plate of the waffle maker and spread it evenly to cover the plate properly
5. Sprinkle the sliced olives as per choice over the mixture and close the lid
6. Cook for at least 4 minutes to get the desired crunch
7. Remove the chaffle from the heat
8. Make as many chaffles as your mixture and waffle maker allow
9. Serve hot and enjoy!

Cauliflower Mozzarella Chaffle

Preparation time:

15 minutes

Cooking time:

8 minutes

Servings: 2

Ingredients:

- Cauliflower: 1 cup
- Egg: 2
- Mozzarella cheese: 1 cup and 4 tbsp
- Tomato sauce: 6 tbsp
- Basil: ½ tsp
- Garlic: ½ tbsp
- Butter: 1 tsp

Directions:

1. In a pan, add butter and include small pieces of cauliflower to it
2. Stir for two minutes and then add garlic and basil
3. Set aside the cooked cauliflower
4. Preheat the mini waffle maker if needed
5. Mix cooked cauliflower, eggs, and 1 cup mozzarella cheese properly
6. Spread it to the mini waffle maker thoroughly
7. Cook for 4 minutes or till it turns crispy and then remove it from the waffle maker

8. Make as many mini chaffles as you can
9. Now in a baking tray, line these mini chaffles and top with the tomato sauce and grated mozzarella cheese
10. Put the tray in the oven at 400 degrees until the cheese melts
11. Serve hot

Plain Artichok Chaffle

Preparation time:

10 minutes

Cooking time:

5 minutes

Servings: 2

Ingredients:

- Artichokes: 1 cup chopped
- Egg: 1
- Mozzarella cheese: 1/2 cup (shredded)
- Cream cheese: 1 ounce
- Salt: as per your taste
- Garlic powder: ¼ tsp

Directions:

1. Preheat a mini waffle maker if needed and grease it
2. In a mixing bowl, add all the ingredients
3. Mix them all well
4. Pour the mixture to the lower plate of the waffle maker and spread it evenly to cover the plate properly
5. Close the lid
6. Cook for at least 4 minutes to get the desired crunch
7. Remove the chaffle from the heat and keep aside for around one minute

8. Make as many chaffles as your mixture and waffle maker allow
9. Serve hot with your favorite keto sauce

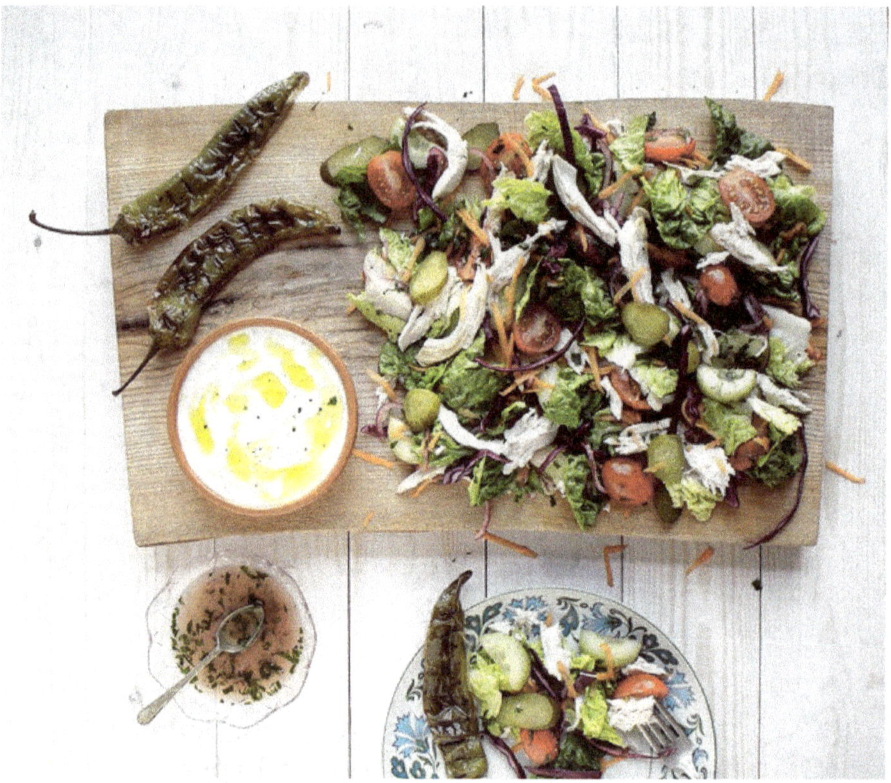

Pecan Pie Cake Chaffle:

Preparation Time:

15 minutes

Cooking Time:

25 minutes

Servings: 2

Ingredients:

- For Pecan Pie Chaffle:
- Egg: 1
- Cream cheese: 2 tbsp
- Maple extract: ½ tbsp
- Almond flour: 4 tbsp
- Sukrin Gold: 1 tbsp
- Baking powder: ½ tbsp
- Pecan: 2 tbsp chopped
- Heavy whipping cream: 1 tbsp
- For Pecan Pie Filling:
- Butter: 2 tbsp
- Sukrin Gold: 1 tbsp
- Pecan: 2 tbsp chopped
- Heavy whipping cream: 2 tbsp
- Maple syrup: 2 tbsp
- Egg yolk: 2 large
- Salt: a pinch

Directions:

1. In a small saucepan, add sweetener, butter, syrups, and heavy whipping cream and use a low flame to heat
2. Mix all the ingredients well together

3. Remove from heat and add egg yolks and mix
4. Now put it on heat again and stir
5. Add pecan and salt to the mixture and let it simmer
6. It will thicken then remove from heat and let it rest
7. For the chaffles, add all the ingredients except pecans and blend
8. Now add pecan with a spoon
9. Preheat a mini waffle maker if needed and grease it
10. Pour the mixture to the lower plate of the waffle maker and spread it evenly to cover the plate properly and close the lid
11. Cook for at least 4 minutes to get the desired crunch
12. Remove the chaffle from the heat and keep aside for around one minute
13. Make as many chaffles as your mixture and waffle maker allow
14. Add 1/3 the previously prepared pecan pie filling to the chaffle and arrange like a cake

German Chocolate Chaffle Cake:

Preparation Time:

5 minutes

Cooking Time:

10 minutes

Servings: 2

Ingredients:

- For Chocolate Chaffle:
- Egg: 1
- Cream cheese: 2 tbsp
- Powdered sweetener: 1 tbsp
- Vanilla extract: ½ tbsp
- Instant coffee powder: ¼ tsp
- Almond flour: 1 tbsp
- Cocoa powder: 1 tbsp (unsweetened)
- For Filling:
- Egg Yolk: 1
- Heavy cream: ¼ cup
- Butter: 1 tbsp
- Powdered sweetener: 2 tbsp
- Caramel: ½ tsp
- Coconut flakes: ¼ cup
- Coconut flour: 1 tsp
- Pecans: ¼ cups chopped

Directions:

1. Preheat a mini waffle maker if needed and grease it
2. In a mixing bowl, beat eggs and add the remaining chaffle ingredients

3. Mix them all well
4. Pour the mixture to the lower plate of the waffle maker and spread it evenly to cover the plate properly and close the lid
5. Cook for at least 4 minutes to get the desired crunch
6. Remove the chaffle from the heat and let them cool completely
7. Make as many chaffles as your mixture and waffle maker allow
8. In a small pan, mix heavy cream, egg yolk, sweetener, and butter at low heat for around 5 minutes
9. Remove from heat and add the remaining ingredients to make the filling
10. Stack chaffles on one another and add filling in between to enjoy the cake

Almond Chocolate Chaffle Cake:

Preparation Time:

5 minutes

Cooking Time:

10 minutes

Servings: 2

Ingredients:

- For Chocolate Chaffle:
- Egg: 1
- Cream cheese: 2 tbsp
- Powdered sweetener: 1 tbsp
- Vanilla extract: ½ tbsp
- Instant coffee powder: ¼ tsp
- Almond flour: 1 tbsp
- Cocoa powder: 1 tbsp (unsweetened)
- For Coconut Filling:
- Melted Coconut Oil: 1 ½ tbsp
- Heavy cream: 1 tbsp
- Cream cheese: 4 tbsp
- Powdered sweetener: 1 tbsp
- Vanilla extract: ½ tbsp
- Coconut: ¼ cup finely shredded
- Whole almonds: 14

Directions:

1. Preheat a mini waffle maker if needed and grease it
2. In a mixing bowl, add all the chaffle ingredients
3. Mix them all well

4. Pour the mixture to the lower plate of the waffle maker and spread it evenly to cover the plate properly
5. Close the lid
6. Cook for at least 4 minutes to get the desired crunch
7. Remove the chaffle from the heat and keep aside for around one minute
8. Make as many chaffles as your mixture and waffle maker allow
9. Except for almond, add all the filling ingredients in a bowl and mix well
10. Spread the filling on the chaffle and spread almonds on top with another chaffle at almonds – stack the chaffles and fillings like a cake and enjoy

Carrot Cake Chaffle

Preparation Time:

10 minutes

Cooking Time:

15 minutes

Servings: 2

Ingredients:

- For Carrot Chaffle Cake:
- Carrot: ½ cup (shredded)
- Egg: 1
- Heavy whipping cream: 2 tbsp
- Butter: 2 tbsp (melted)
- Powdered sweetener: 2 tbsp
- Walnuts: 1 tbsp (chopped)
- Almond flour: ¾ cup
- Cinnamon powder: 2 tsp
- Baking powder: 1 tsp
- Pumpkin sauce: 1 tsp
- For Cream Cheese Frosting:
- Cream cheese: ½ cup
- Heavy whipping cream: 2 tbsp
- Vanilla extract: 1 tsp
- Powdered sweetener: ¼ cup

Directions:

1. Mix all the ingredients together one by one until they form a uniform consistency
2. Preheat a mini waffle maker if needed and grease it

3. Pour the mixture to the lower plate of the waffle maker
4. Close the lid
5. Cook for at least 4 minutes to get the desired crunch
6. Prepare frosting by combining all the ingredients of the cream cheese frosting using a hand mixer
7. Remove the chaffle from the heat and keep aside for around a few minutes
8. Make as many chaffles as your mixture and waffle maker allow
9. Stack the chaffles with frosting in between in such a way that it gives the look of a cake

Peanut Butter Keto Chaffle Cake

Preparation Time:

5 minutes

Cooking Time:

10 minutes

Servings: 2

Ingredients:

- For Chaffles:
- Egg: 1
- Peanut Butter:: 2 tbsp (sugar-free)
- Monkfruit: 2 tbsp
- Baking powder: ¼ tsp
- Peanut butter extract: ¼ tsp
- Heavy whipping cream: 1 tsp
- For Peanut Butter Frosting:
- Monkfruit: 2 tsp
- Cream cheese: 2 tbsp
- Butter: 1 tbsp
- Peanut butter: 1 tbsp (sugar-free)
- Vanilla: ¼ tsp

Directions:

1. Preheat a mini waffle maker if needed and grease it
2. In a mixing bowl, beat eggs and add all the chaffle ingredients
3. Mix them all well and pour the mixture to the lower plate of the waffle maker
4. Close the lid

5. Cook for at least 4 minutes to get the desired crunch
6. Remove the chaffle from the heat and keep aside for around a few minutes
7. Make as many chaffles as your mixture and waffle maker allow
8. In a separate bowl, add all the frosting ingredients and whisk well to give it a uniform consistency
9. Assemble chaffles in a way that in between two chaffles you put the frosting and make the cake

Strawberry Shortcake Chaffle

Preparation Time:

5 minutes

Cooking Time:

10 minutes

Servings: 2

Ingredients:

- Egg: 1
- Heavy Whipping Cream: 1 tbsp
- Any non-sugar sweetener: 2 tbsp
- Coconut Flour: 1 tsp
- Cake batter extract: ½ tsp
- Baking powder: ¼ tsp
- Strawberry: 4 or as per your taste

Directions:

1. Preheat a mini waffle maker if needed and grease it
2. In a mixing bowl, beat eggs and add non-sugar sweetener, coconut flour, baking powder, and cake batter extract
3. Mix them all well and pour the mixture to the lower plate of the waffle maker
4. Close the lid
5. Cook for at least 4 minutes to get the desired crunch
6. Remove the chaffle from the heat and keep aside for around two minutes

7. Make as many chaffles as your mixture and waffle maker allow
8. Serve with whipped cream and strawberries on top

Italian Cream Chaffle Cake

Preparation Time:

8 minutes

Cooking Time:

12 minutes

Servings: 3

Ingredients:

- For Chaffle:
- Egg: 4
- Mozzarella Cheese: ½ cup
- Almond flour: 1 tbsp
- Coconut flour: 4 tbsp
- Monkfruit sweetener: 1 tbsp
- Vanilla extract: 1 tsp
- Baking powder: 1 ½ tsp
- Cinnamon powder: ½ tsp
- Butter: 1 tbsp (melted)
- Coconut: 1 tsp (shredded)
- Walnuts: 1 tsp (chopped)
- For Italian Cream Frosting:
- Cream cheese: 4 tbsp
- Butter: 2 tbsp
- Vanilla: ½ tsp
- Monkfruit sweetener: 2 tbs

Directions:

1. Blend eggs, cream cheese, sweetener, vanilla, coconut flour, melted butter, almond flour, and baking powder

2. Make the mixture creamy
3. Preheat a mini waffle maker if needed and grease it
4. Pour the mixture to the lower plate of the waffle maker
5. Close the lid
6. Cook for at least 4 minutes to get the desired crunch
7. Remove the chaffle from the heat and keep aside to cool it
8. Make as many chaffles as your mixture and waffle maker allow
9. Garnish with shredded coconut and chopped walnuts

Banana Cake Pudding Chaffle

Preparation Time:

10 minutes

Cooking Time:

1 hour

Servings: 2

Ingredients:

- For Banana Chaffle:
- Cream cheese: 2 tbsp
- Banana extract: 1 tsp
- Mozzarella cheese: ¼ cup
- Egg: 1
- Sweetener: 2 tbsp
- Almond flour: 4 tbsp
- Baking powder: 1 tsp
- For Banana Pudding:
- Egg yolk: 1 large
- Powdered sweetener: 3 tbsp
- Xanthan gum: ½ tsp
- Heavy whipping cream: 1/2 cup
- Banana extract: ½ tsp
- Salt: a pinch

Directions:

1. In a pan, add powdered sweetener, heavy cream, and egg yolk and whisk continuously so the mixture thickens
2. Simmer for a minute only

3. Add xanthan gum to the mixture and whisk again
4. Remove the pan from heat and add banana extract and salt and mix them all well
5. Shift the mixture to a glass dish and refrigerate the pudding
6. Preheat a mini waffle maker if needed and grease it
7. In a mixing bowl, add all the chaffle ingredients
8. Mix them all well and pour the mixture to the lower plate of the waffle maker
9. Close the lid
10. Cook for at least 5 minutes to get the desired crunch
11. Remove the chaffle from the heat and keep aside for around a few minutes
12. Stack chaffles and pudding one by one to form a cake

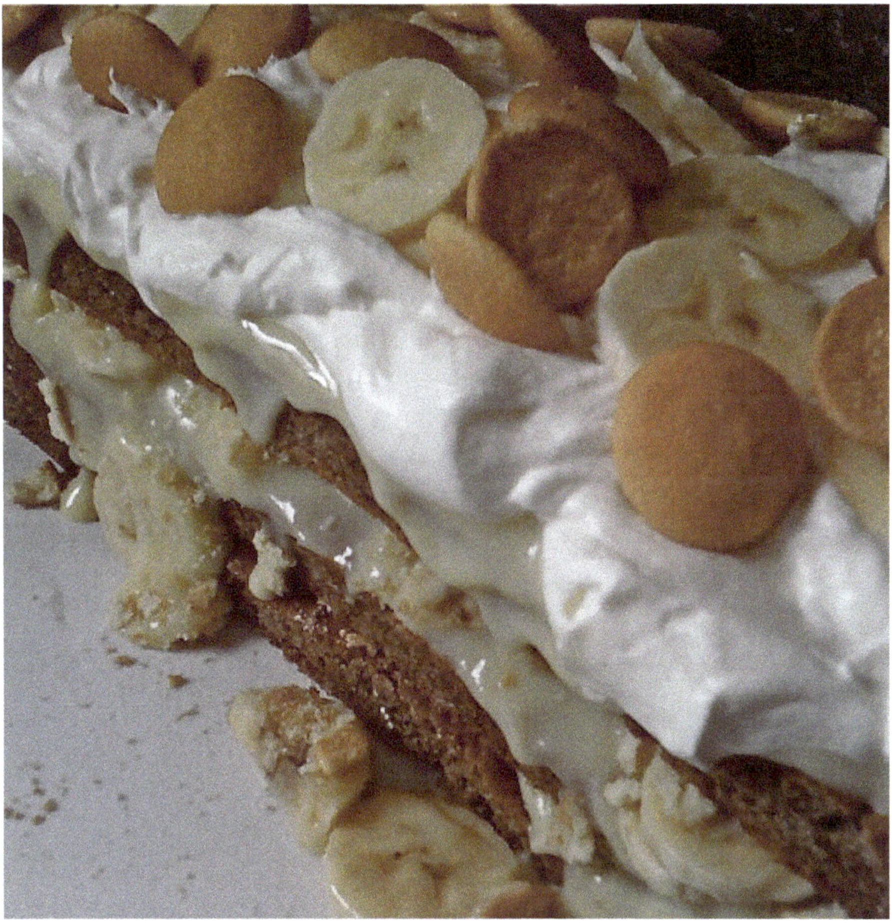

CPSIA information can be obtained
at www.ICGtesting.com
Printed in the USA
BVHW091110210621
610125BV00003B/451

9 781803 177809